Herniated Disc

A Beginner's Quick Start Guide to Managing the Condition Through Diet and Other Natural Methods, With Sample Curated Recipes

mf

copyright © 2022 Patrick Marshwell

All rights reserved No part of this book may be reproduced, or stored in a retrieval system, or transmitted in any form or by any means, electronic, mechanical, photocopying, recording, or otherwise, without express written permission of the publisher.

Disclaimer

By reading this disclaimer, you are accepting the terms of the disclaimer in full. If you disagree with this disclaimer, please do not read the guide.

All of the content within this guide is provided for informational and educational purposes only, and should not be accepted as independent medical or other professional advice. The author is not a doctor, physician, nurse, mental health provider, or registered nutritionist/dietician. Therefore, using and reading this guide does not establish any form of a physician-patient relationship.

Always consult with a physician or another qualified health provider with any issues or questions you might have regarding any sort of medical condition. Do not ever disregard any qualified professional medical advice or delay seeking that advice because of anything you have read in this guide. The information in this guide is not intended to be any sort of medical advice and should not be used in lieu of any medical advice by a licensed and qualified medical professional.

The information in this guide has been compiled from a variety of known sources. However, the author cannot attest to or guarantee the accuracy of each source and thus should not be held liable for any errors or omissions.

You acknowledge that the publisher of this guide will not be held liable for any loss or damage of any kind incurred as a result of this guide or the reliance on any information provided within this guide. You acknowledge and agree that you assume all risk and responsibility for any action you undertake in response to the information in this guide.

Using this guide does not guarantee any particular result (e.g., weight loss or a cure). By reading this guide, you acknowledge that there are no guarantees to any specific outcome or results you can expect.

All product names, diet plans, or names used in this guide are for identification purposes only and are the property of their respective owners. The use of these names does not imply endorsement. All other trademarks cited herein are the property of their respective owners.

Where applicable, this guide is not intended to be a substitute for the original work of this diet plan and is, at most, a supplement to the original work for this diet plan and never a direct substitute. This guide is a personal expression of the facts of that diet plan.

Where applicable, persons shown in the cover images are stock photography models and the publisher has obtained the rights to use the images through license agreements with third-party stock image companies.

Table of Contents

Introduction	6
What Are the Symptoms of Herniated Discs?	8
What Causes Herniated Discs?	10
How Are Herniated Discs Diagnosed?	12
What Are the Complications of Herniated Discs?	14
How Are Herniated Discs Treated?	16
How Can You Prevent Herniated Discs?	18
Managing Herniated Discs Through Natural Methods	22
Managing Herniated Discs Through Diet and Nutrition	25
Foods to Eat	25
Foods to Avoid	28
Sample Recipes	31
Baked Flounder	32
Salmon with Avocados and Brussels Sprouts	33
Asian-Themed Macrobiotic Bowl	36
Chicken Salad	38
Baked Salmon	39
Asian Zucchini Salad	40
Low FODMAP Burger	41
Stir-Fried Cabbage and Apples	42
Asparagus and Greens Salad with Tahini and Poppy Seed Dressing	43
Stir-Fried Cabbage and Apples	44
Roasted Chicken Thighs	45
Arugula and Mushroom Salad	46
Cauliflower and Mushroom Bake	47
Fresh Asparagus Salad	48
Detox Bowl	50
Conclusion	52
References and Helpful Links	54

Introduction

Discs protect the bones (vertebrae) that make up the spine in the back. These discs are round, like small pillows, and have a tough outer layer (annulus) that surrounds the nucleus. Discs are made of cartilage and are between each of the vertebrae in the spine. They function as shock absorbers for the vertebrae.

A herniated disc also called a bulged, slipped, or ruptured disc happens when a piece of the disc nucleus is pushed through a tear or break in the annulus and into the spinal canal. When a disc bulges, it is usually in the early stages of wearing out. The spinal canal is small, which does not have enough room for the spinal nerve and the herniated disc fragment that has moved. Because of this, the disc pushes on the spinal nerves, which can cause pain that can be very bad.

Most herniated discs happen in the lower back, and they are induced by wear and tear that comes with age. But any disc in your spine can pop out of place. Some individuals are born with spinal canals that are narrower than normal or with other problems that make them more likely to have a herniated disc.

Most herniated discs happen when someone lifts something heavy or goes through a traumatic event like a car crash. A herniated disc is also common because of the wear and tear that comes with getting older.

Most of the time, a herniated disc is treated conservatively with over-the-counter pain relievers, anti-inflammatory drugs, ice packs, and heat therapy. Physical therapy may also be suggested to help stretch and strengthen the muscles that support your spine. If conservative treatments don't help alleviate your pain or if your herniated disc is making your arms or legs weak, numb, or tingle, you may need surgery to remove the damaged part of the disc and relieve the pressure on your nerves.

In this quick start guide, we'll discuss the following in detail:

- What are the symptoms of herniated discs?
- What causes herniated discs?
- How is it diagnosed?
- What are the complications of herniated discs?
- What are the medical treatments for herniated discs?
- How can you prevent herniated discs?
- Managing herniated discs through natural methods
- Managing herniated discs through diet

Keep reading to learn everything you need to know about managing herniated discs through diet and other natural methods!

What Are the Symptoms of Herniated Discs?

Not all herniated discs will cause symptoms. Small herniated discs often do not cause any pain because they do not put pressure on the spinal cord or nerves. The location of the herniated disc also determines whether or not a person will experience symptoms. A herniated disc in the lower back is more likely to cause symptoms than a herniated disc in the neck.

If you experience one or more of the following symptoms, you may have a herniated disc:

Sciatica

This is the most common symptom of a herniated disc. Sciatica is pain that radiates from your lower back down your leg. The pain may be sharp or dull. It may feel like a burning sensation or a numbing sensation. You may also have tingling, weakness, or numbness in your leg or foot.

Low back pain

Low back pain is a common symptom of a herniated disc. When a disc herniates, the inner gelatinous material leaks out and puts pressure on the adjacent nerve root. This can cause pain, numbness, or weakness in the affected area. You may feel a dull ache in your lower back. The pain may be worse when you sit or stand for long periods. You may also have pain when you cough or sneeze.

Arm or leg pain

You may feel pain, numbness, or tingling in your arm or leg. The pain may be worse when you move your arm or leg.

Neck pain

You may feel pain in your neck, shoulders, or arms. The pain may be worse when you move your head or neck.

Headache

You may have a headache at the base of your skull. The headache may be worse when you bend your head forward.

These are the most common symptoms of a herniated disc. If you experience any of these symptoms, you should see a doctor.

What Causes Herniated Discs?

A herniated disc occurs when the outer layer of the disc ruptures, allowing the inner gel-like substance to leak out. This can happen due to several different causes, including trauma, degenerative changes, and aging.

Age

Herniated discs are caused by wear and tear that comes with age. The discs in your spine act as shock absorbers. They cushion the vertebrae and allow the spine to move. Over time, the discs begin to break down and lose their ability to cushion the vertebrae. This can cause the discs to bulge or herniation.

Lifting something heavy

One of the most common causes of a herniated disc is lifting something heavy. When you lift something, your spine bears the brunt of the weight. If you try to lift something too heavy or use the incorrect form, you can put too much pressure on your discs, causing them to rupture.

Traumatic events

A traumatic event like a car accident can cause the discs in your spine to bulge or herniation.

Narrow spinal canal

Some people are born with a spinal canal that is narrower than normal. This can make it more likely for the discs in their spine to bulge or herniation.

Other causes of a herniated disc include repetitive motions, obesity, and smoking. These activities can all lead to degenerative changes in the discs, making them more susceptible to rupture.

Ultimately, a herniated disc can be caused by a variety of different factors. However, understanding the causes can help you take steps to prevent this condition from developing in the first place.

How Are Herniated Discs Diagnosed?

A herniated disc is most often diagnosed with a physical exam and review of your medical history. Your doctor will ask about your symptoms and how long you've been experiencing them. He or she will also ask about your medical history, including any previous injuries to your spine.

To help confirm the diagnosis, your doctor may order one or more imaging tests. These can include an X-ray, MRI, or CT scan.

X-ray

This can help show if there is any damage to the bones in your spine.

CT scan

A CT scan also uses special X-ray equipment, but it takes several pictures from different angles. This can help show the discs in your spine and if they are bulging or herniated.

MRI

An MRI uses powerful magnets and radio waves to create detailed images of your spine. This can help show the discs in your spine and if they are bulging or herniated.

Electromyogram (EMG)

Your doctor may also order an electromyogram (EMG) to test the nerves in your arms or legs.

By understanding the symptoms and how the spine works, doctors can accurately diagnose a herniated disc and create a treatment plan that will help the patient find relief. These imaging tests can help confirm the diagnosis and guide further treatment. If you have a herniated disc, you may need to see a spine specialist for additional treatment.

What Are the Complications of Herniated Discs?

Herniated discs are a common, yet serious, condition that can cause a variety of complications. If you have a herniated disc, it is important to seek treatment right away to prevent these complications from occurring.

Nerve damage

One complication that can result from a herniated disc is nerve damage. When the disc presses on the nerves in your spine, it can cause permanent damage. This can lead to pain, numbness, and weakness in the affected area. In severe cases, it can even cause paralysis.

Spinal cord injury

When the disc presses on the spinal cord, it can cause paralysis. This can lead to a loss of sensation and muscle control in the affected area. In severe cases, it can even result in death.

Loss of bowel or bladder control

Herniated discs can also cause bladder and bowel incontinence. When the disc presses on the nerves that control these functions, it can disrupt their normal functioning.

Arthritis

Herniated discs can also lead to arthritis. The inflammation and damage caused by the herniated disc can put pressure on joints and wear down cartilage, leading to pain and stiffness.

While most people with herniated discs do not experience any complications, it is important to be aware of the potential risks associated with this condition.

How Are Herniated Discs Treated?

The treatment for herniated discs depends on the severity of your symptoms. If you have mild symptoms, your doctor may recommend that you take over-the-counter pain relievers and rest. If you have severe symptoms, your doctor may recommend one or more of the following treatments:

Physical therapy

One treatment option for herniated discs is physical therapy. Physical therapy uses different exercises and stretches to help ease the pain and promote healing. Generally, a course of physical therapy will last for several weeks. The therapist will work with the patient to gradually increase the intensity of the exercises as the patient's condition improves.

Physical therapy can be an effective treatment for herniated discs, and it often leads to long-term relief from pain. However, it is important to note that physical therapy is not a cure for herniated discs. In some cases, the disc may need to be surgically removed to provide relief from pain.

Epidural steroid injections

Epidural steroid injection (ESI) involves injecting steroids directly into the epidural space surrounding the spinal cord. ESI is generally considered to be a safe and effective treatment for herniated discs, with a success rate of approximately 50-80%.

It is important to note, however, that ESI is not a cure for herniated discs and does not always provide long-term relief. In some cases, multiple injections may be necessary to achieve the desired effect.

Surgery

If conservative treatments don't work, your doctor may recommend surgery. Although it is invasive, surgery is often successful in relieving pain and restoring function. The surgeon will make an incision in the back and remove the herniated disc.

In some cases, a small portion of the disc may be removed. In other cases, the entire disc may be removed. In either case, the surgeon will then fuse the vertebrae to stabilize the spine. This procedure is usually effective in relieving pain and restoring function.

However, it is important to note that it is also associated with a risk of complications, such as infection and nerve damage. As with any surgery, you should discuss the risks and benefits with your doctor before making a decision.

How Can You Prevent Herniated Discs?

Back pain is something that affects a significant portion of the population at some time in their life. Herniated discs are a major source of back pain and are one of the most common causes. When the pliable, inner material of a disc escapes via a tear in the tougher outer layer, this is known as a herniated disc.

This can cause the spinal nerves to get compressed, which can result in pain as well as other symptoms. You may assist avoid herniated discs by doing several different things, including the following:

Exercising

It is essential to engage in regular physical activity and keep healthy body weight to reduce the risk of experiencing a herniated disc. The spine may be supported better and the strain on the discs can be relieved with the aid of exercises that strengthen the abdomen and back muscles.

In addition, stretching exercises can assist in developing flexibility and lower the risk of injury. If you have a history of back problems or are at risk of developing new ones, you should steer clear of high-impact activities like jogging.

Maintaining a healthy weight

Keeping a healthy weight is one of the finest things you can do to protect yourself from getting a herniated disc. Discs are meant to act as a cushion between the vertebrae and absorb shocks, but if they are consistently subjected to tension, they run the risk of becoming injured.

When the tissue of a disc begins to deteriorate, it may bulge or burst, resulting in discomfort and maybe damaged nerves. Extra weight places additional strain on the discs, which can contribute to the development of herniation. You may assist in lowering the risk of herniated discs by ensuring that your weight is kept at a healthy level.

Using proper lifting techniques

When picking up something heavy, ensure that you bend at the knees rather than the back and keep your back in a straight position. When lifting, try to avoid twisting your body in any way. Your spine will feel less pressure as a result of this.

Maintaining a good posture

Maintaining correct posture helps to ensure that your body weight is distributed evenly throughout your spine. Try to avoid sitting in one posture for an extended period or slouching. Take frequent breaks to move around, stretch, and stroll about the area.

Wearing comfortable shoes

It is imperative to take every precaution possible to avoid herniated discs since they can cause excruciating pain and should be avoided at all costs. Wearing comfy shoes is one of the most effective strategies to accomplish this goal. Shoes that offer a high level of support can alleviate some of the pressure that is placed on the spine, which in turn can assist in lessening the risk of discs being herniated.

Make sure your workstation is ergonomic

If your job requires you to sit for extended periods, you should make sure your workspace is comfortable. Your chances of getting a herniated disc might be lowered further if you give yourself frequent opportunities to get up and walk around.

Eating a healthy diet

Maintaining a healthy weight with the support of nutritious food helps to reduce the amount of pressure that is placed on the spine. Eating a diet rich in fruits and vegetables and consuming an adequate amount of calcium can also contribute to the maintenance of healthy bones.

Herniated discs are a rather frequent ailment that can produce discomfort in addition to other symptoms. There are several different treatment options accessible to those who suffer from herniated discs. The majority of persons who have herniated discs can experience alleviation from their symptoms with the use of appropriate therapy.

Managing Herniated Discs Through Natural Methods

There are several things you can do to manage your herniated discs through diet and other natural methods.

Diet

Eating a healthy diet is important for managing herniated discs. Some foods that may help reduce inflammation include omega-3 fatty acids, turmeric, and ginger.

Exercise

Exercise helps to strengthen the muscles around your spine, which can help to avoid injury. However, be sure to avoid high-impact activities such as running if you are at risk for a disc injury.

Yoga

Yoga can help to decompress the spine and stretch the muscles around the discs. This can help to reduce pain and improve the range of motion. In addition, yoga can help to strengthen the core muscles, which can provide support for the spine and help to prevent future herniated discs. If you are experiencing pain from a herniated disc, talk to your doctor about whether yoga may be right for you.

Acupuncture

Acupuncture is a traditional Chinese medicine technique that involves inserting thin needles into the skin at specific points. It is thought to help reduce pain by releasing endorphins and other chemicals in the brain.

Massage

Massage can help reduce pain and muscle tension.

Chiropractic care

Chiropractic care is a type of alternative medicine that focuses on the diagnosis and treatment of musculoskeletal disorders. Chiropractors use a variety of techniques to manipulate the spine and other joints in the body.

Herbal remedies

A herniated disc can be a painful and debilitating condition. Fortunately, several natural methods can help to reduce inflammation and pain. These include Boswellia, willow bark, and Devil's claw.

Boswellia is an herb that has been used for centuries in traditional Indian medicine. It is thought to help reduce inflammation by inhibiting the production of leukotrienes, substances that contribute to inflammation.

Willow bark is another herbal remedy that has been used for centuries to relieve pain. It contains salicin, a compound that is transformed into salicylic acid in the body, which is then thought to block pain signals.

Devil's Claw is a third herbal remedy that is thought to be effective for managing pain associated with herniated discs. It is native to Southern Africa and has been used traditionally to treat pain and inflammation. It can be effective in reducing pain and improving function in people with herniated discs.

Herniated discs can be a painful condition. However, there are several things you can do to manage your symptoms through diet, exercise, and other natural methods. With proper treatment, most people with herniated discs can find relief from their symptoms.

Managing Herniated Discs Through Diet and Nutrition

What you eat can have a big impact on herniated discs and other spine conditions. Eating a healthy diet is important for managing herniated discs.

Foods to Eat

Omega-3 fatty acids, turmeric, and ginger are examples of some of the foods that have the potential to help decrease inflammation. The maintenance of a healthy spine also requires taking dietary supplements, particularly those rich in calcium, iron, phosphorus, vitamin D, and magnesium.

Omega-3 fatty acids

It is well-established that omega-3 fatty acids can aid in the reduction of inflammation, which, in turn, can assist in alleviating pain and other symptoms. Nuts and seeds, in addition to fatty fish such as salmon and tuna, are examples of foods that are high in omega-3 fatty acids. If you suffer from a herniated disc, including these items in your diet may help to alleviate some of the associated pain and other symptoms.

Turmeric

Curcumin, a molecule that is known to have anti-inflammatory qualities, may be found in the spice turmeric, which bears the same name. In addition, turmeric has been shown to assist in enhancing circulation and may also aid in promoting joint flexibility. As a consequence of this, it has the potential to be helpful for those who have herniated discs.

Ginger

Ginger is a kind of root that is believed to have anti-inflammatory characteristics. These features may help alleviate the discomfort that is linked with herniated discs. Fresh, dried, or powdered forms, as well as oil, are all viable means of consumption.

Calcium

Calcium plays a crucial role in the upkeep of healthy bones. It may also assist in lowering one's likelihood of getting osteoporosis, which is a disorder that results in the bones becoming fragile and porous. Postmenopausal women, who are at a greater risk of developing osteoporosis, should pay extra attention to making sure they get an adequate amount of calcium in their diet.

Iron

Hemoglobin is a protein that is responsible for transporting oxygen throughout the body, and the creation of hemoglobin requires the mineral iron. Additionally, it is necessary for the formation of healthy bones as well as their continued upkeep. Those who suffer from herniated discs could find relief from an increase in their iron consumption.

Phosphorus

A mineral known as phosphorus may be found in every one of the body's cells. In addition to playing a role in the growth and repair of tissues, it is necessary for the generation of energy in the body. Phosphorus is present in a variety of foods, including meat, chicken, fish, eggs, and dairy goods and products.

Vitamin D

Calcium and phosphorus can only be absorbed into the body if vitamin D is present. It is also believed to contribute to the preservation of bone health in the body. Milk and orange juice may be supplemented with vitamin D, and some fatty fish, such as salmon, are natural sources of the vitamin.

Magnesium

In the human body, the mineral magnesium plays an important role in more than 300 different metabolic activities. It is essential for the growth and preservation of bones, as well as for the function of nerves and muscles. Nuts, vegetables with dark green leafy parts, and whole grains are good sources of magnesium.

Foods to Avoid

Some meals can assist in the management of the symptoms of a herniated disc, but there are also certain foods that you should try to stay away from. Foods that fall into this category include those that are heavy in sugar, salt, and fat. You should also steer clear of beverages containing alcohol and caffeine.

Sugary foods

It has been established that eating foods high in sugar can contribute to inflammation. Since inflammation is one of the leading causes of herniated discs, it stands to reason that avoiding foods high in sugar can assist in minimizing the chance of developing this condition. In addition to this, they can also cause weight gain, which places more strain on the spine and can exacerbate back problems.

Salt

The use of salt can raise the risk of being dehydrated and make it more challenging for the body to absorb nutrients that are necessary for proper functioning. In addition, consuming an excessive amount of salt can cause the body to retain water, which can result in inflammation as well as pain. It is in your best interest to steer clear of processed meals because they typically include a lot of salt.

Fatty foods

Consuming foods high in fat and calories, such as fatty meals, can lead to weight gain. They are also capable of causing inflammation, which, in turn, can exacerbate the discomfort that is caused by herniated discs. It is in your best interest to steer clear of meals that are fried, meats that have been processed, and full-fat dairy products.

Alcohol

Consumption of alcohol has been associated with an increased risk of getting herniated discs. This is probably because drinking alcohol can contribute to dehydration, which in turn can promote inflammation.

Caffeine

It has been shown that caffeine use increases the chance of being dehydrated, which can then contribute to inflammation. Additionally, caffeine has been shown to inhibit the body's ability to absorb calcium, which is an essential mineral for maintaining healthy bones and teeth. It is recommended that you consume no more than 200 milligrams of caffeine each day.

It is essential to maintain a healthy diet if you have herniated discs in your back. It's possible that eating foods like omega-3 fatty acids, turmeric, and ginger might be good for your health if they help reduce inflammation. You should also stay away from meals high in sugar, salt, and fat, as well as alcoholic beverages and caffeine. It is essential to treat the symptoms of a herniated disc by adhering to a healthy diet and keeping a healthy weight to manage the condition.

Sample Recipes

Baked Flounder

Ingredients:

- 1 lb. flounder, fileted
- 1/4 tsp. salt
- 1 cup halved red grapes
- 1 tbsp. extra-virgin olive oil
- 2 tbsp. parsley, chopped finely
- 1 tbsp. lemon juice
- 1 cup almonds, chopped and toasted
- freshly ground black pepper, to taste

Instructions:

1. Preheat the oven to 375°F.
2. Place fish on a sheet tray. Season with olive oil, salt, and pepper.
3. Combine the almonds, grapes, lemon juice, parsley, 1-1/2 tsp. of olive oil, 1/8 tsp of salt, and black pepper in a bowl.
4. Bake the fish for about 3 minutes.
5. Flip the fish and return to the oven.
6. Bake for another 3 minutes, or until the fish is starting to flake, while the center is still translucent. Don't overcook.
7. Serve immediately, topped with the grape mixture.

Salmon with Avocados and Brussels Sprouts

Ingredients:

- 2 lbs. of salmon filet, divided into 4 pieces
- 1 tsp. ground cumin
- 1 tsp. onion powder
- 1 tsp. paprika powder
- 1/2 tsp. garlic powder
- 1 tsp. chili powder
- Himalayan sea salt
- black pepper, freshly ground

Avocado sauce:

- 2 chopped avocados
- 1 lime, squeezed for the juice
- 1 tbsp. extra-virgin olive oil
- 1 tbsp. fresh minced cilantro
- 1 diced small red onion
- 1 minced garlic clove
- Himalayan sea salt to taste
- black pepper, freshly ground

Brussels sprouts:

- 3 lbs. of Brussels sprouts
- 1/2 cup raw honey
- 1/2 cup balsamic vinegar
- 1/2 cup melted coconut oil

- 1 cup dried cranberries
- Himalayan sea salt
- black pepper, freshly ground

Instructions:

To make the salmon and avocado sauce:

1. Combine cumin, onion, chili powder, garlic, and paprika seasoned with salt and pepper. Mix well before dry rubbing on the salmon.
2. Place the salmon in the fridge for 30 minutes.
3. Preheat the grill.
4. In a bowl, mash avocado until the texture becomes smooth. Pour in all the remaining ingredients and mix thoroughly.
5. Grill salmon for 5 minutes on each side or until cooked.
6. Drizzle avocado on cooked salmon.

To prepare the Brussels sprouts:

1. Preheat the oven to 375°F.
2. Mix Brussels sprouts with coconut oil. Season with salt and pepper.
3. Place vegetables on a baking sheet and roast for about 30 minutes.
4. In a separate pan, combine vinegar and honey.

5. Simmer in slow heat until it boils and thickens.
6. Drizzle them on top of the Brussels sprouts.
7. Serve with the salmon.

Asian-Themed Macrobiotic Bowl

Ingredients:

- 2 cups cooked quinoa
- 4 carrots
- 1 package of smoked tofu
- 1 tbsp. nutritional yeast
- 2 tbsp. coconut aminos
- 4 tbsp. sunflower sprouts
- 2 tbsp. fermented vegetables
- 1 cup of shiitake mushrooms
- 1 avocado
- 2 tbsp. hemp seeds
- 2-3 cooked beets
- coconut oil cooking spray

Dressing:

- 2 tbsp. miso paste
- 1 tbsp. tahini
- 1 tbsp. olive oil
- 1/2 lime, juiced
- 3 tbsp. water

Instructions:

1. Roast the carrots in the oven at 400°F for 30-40 minutes.

2. Wash the vegetables, trim them, and spray them with coconut oil.
3. Add them in the oven. When they are cooked, set aside till you are ready to assemble the Buddha bowl.
4. Make the dressing by combining all of the ingredients in a medium-size bowl. If the dressing appears lumpy, add more water.
5. To build the bowl, put the quinoa on the bottom and then arrange the vegetables on top.
6. Sprinkle the bowls with hemp seeds and drizzle the dressing over top.
7. Now serve and enjoy!

Chicken Salad

Ingredients:

- 1 small can premium chunk chicken breast packed in water
- 1 stalk celery, large, finely chopped
- 1/4 cup reduced-fat mayonnaise
- 4 romaine leaves or red leaf lettuce, washed and trimmed
- 8 pcs. cherry tomatoes or 1 ripe tomato, quartered
- 1 cucumber, small and sliced thinly

Instructions:

1. Drain canned chicken and transfer to a bowl.
2. Put in celery and mayonnaise.
3. Mix lightly. Don't crush the chicken.
4. In a separate shallow bowl, place the lettuce neatly.
5. Add in the chicken salad in the middle
6. Add tomatoes and cucumber slices to the plate.
7. Refrigerate before serving, cover with plastic wrap.

Baked Salmon

Ingredients:

- 2 salmon filets
- 6 cups of fresh spinach
- 2 tsp. coconut oil
- 1/4 tsp. turmeric
- lemon juice
- salt
- pepper

Instructions:

1. Preheat the oven to 400°F.
2. Line a baking dish with parchment paper.
3. Marinate salmon filets in lemon juice, coconut oil, turmeric, salt, and pepper.
4. Let it sit for a few minutes. This may also be done the night before to help the juices and flavor get into the salmon.
5. Once the oven is ready, bake salmon for 15 minutes.
6. Add spinach and cook until ready. Season with salt and pepper to taste.
7. Take salmon out of the oven and put spinach beside it.
8. Serve and enjoy.

Asian Zucchini Salad

Ingredients:

- 1 medium zucchini, sliced thinly into spirals
- 1/3 cup rice vinegar
- 3/4 cup avocado oil
- 1 cup sunflower seeds, shells removed
- 1 lb. cabbage, shredded
- 1 tsp. stevia drops
- 1 cup almonds, sliced

Instructions:

1. Cut the zucchini spirals into smaller parts. Set aside.
2. Put almonds, sunflower seeds, and cabbage in a large bowl. Combine the ingredients well.
3. Add zucchini to the mixture.
4. In a small bowl, mix vinegar, stevia, and oil using a whisk or fork.
5. Pour the vinegar mixture all over the zucchini mixture. Toss well. Make sure everything is covered with the dressing.
6. Refrigerate for 2 hours before serving.

Low FODMAP Burger

Ingredients:

- 1-1/4 lbs. ground pork
- 1/2 tsp. salt
- 1/2 tsp. white pepper
- 1/2 tsp. ground nutmeg
- 1/2 tsp. caraway seeds
- 1/2 tsp. ground ginger

Instructions:

1. Preheat the grill then prepare the patty.
2. Using a small mixing bowl, stir together the salt, pepper, nutmeg, and ginger until fully combined.
3. Place the ground in a large mixing bowl and add the spice mixture.
4. Mix thoroughly until spices are evenly distributed to the pork.
5. Make round, flat burger patties using the palm of your hands.
6. Grill the patties and serve with gluten-free buns and mustard sauce.

Stir-Fried Cabbage and Apples

Ingredients:

- 1 shallot, thinly sliced
- 1/2 apple, cut into cubes
- 1/4 savoy cabbage, sliced thinly into strips
- 3–4 radishes, sliced thinly
- 1/2–1 tsp. coconut oil
- salt, to taste

Instructions:

1. Pour some coconut oil into a wok.
2. Add shallot and cook until translucent.
3. Add the cabbage, radish, and apples to the wok.
4. Stir-fry for about 5 minutes. Don't overcook.
5. Add salt to taste.
6. Serve while warm.

Asparagus and Greens Salad with Tahini and Poppy Seed Dressing

Ingredients:

- 10 to 12 asparagus stalks, washed well and sliced into ribbons
- 5 radishes, washed well, and sliced thinly
- 2 to 3 rainbow carrots, peeled and sliced thinly
- 1 handful wild spinach
- 1 small handful of microgreens, washed well
- 1 small handful of sunflower greens, washed well
- optional: few pieces of chive blossoms

For the dressing:

- 2 tbsp. tahini
- 1 tbsp. poppy seeds
- 1 tbsp. extra-virgin olive oil
- salt
- pepper

Instructions:

1. For the dressing, whisk ingredients together in a small bowl.
2. In a separate bowl, toss salad ingredients in the mixture.
3. Drizzle dressing on salad upon serving.

Stir-Fried Cabbage and Apples

Ingredients:

- 1 shallot, thinly sliced
- 1/2 apple, cut into cubes
- 1/4 savoy cabbage, sliced thinly into strips
- 3–4 radishes, sliced thinly
- 1/2–1 tsp. coconut oil
- salt, to taste

Instructions:

1. Pour some coconut oil into a wok.
2. Add shallot and cook until translucent.
3. Add the cabbage, radish, and apples to the wok.
4. Stir-fry for about 5 minutes. Don't overcook.
5. Add salt to taste.
6. Serve while warm.

Roasted Chicken Thighs

Ingredients:

- 1 tbsp. avocado oil
- 1 pinch Himalayan pink salt
- 4 chicken thighs with skin
- 1 tsp. Primal Palate super gyro seasoning

Instructions:

1. Pour avocado oil over a medium-sized oven-safe pot.
2. Sauté over medium heat for 2 to 3 minutes or until the skins begin to brown.
3. Place the chicken in a large skillet over medium-high heat. Sear for about 2 to 3 minutes for each side, starting with the skin side.
4. Season generously with salt and Primal Palate Super Gyro seasoning.
5. Place the chicken in an oven preheated to 350°F.
6. Bake for one hour while covered.
7. Serve and enjoy.

Arugula and Mushroom Salad

Ingredients:

- 5 oz. arugula washed
- 1 lb. fresh mushrooms
- 1/4 tsp. shoyu
- 1/2 red onion
- 1 tbsp. olive oil
- 1 tbsp. mirin

For tofu cheese:

- 1/8 cup umeboshi vinegar
- .1/2 firm tofu

Instructions:

1. In a bowl, add the rinsed tofu. Crumble and pour in vinegar.
2. In a separate bowl add shoyu, red onions, salt, olive oil, and mirin. 3. Mix to combine.
3. Add in the arugula and toss to combine with the dressing.
4. Serve and enjoy.

Cauliflower and Mushroom Bake

Ingredients:

- 3 cups cauliflower florets
- 1 cup fresh mushroom, chopped
- 1/2 cup red onion, chopped
- 1/3 cup green onion, chopped
- 2 tsp. apple cider vinegar
- 2 tsp. lemon juice
- 1/2 tsp. salt
- 1/4 tsp. pepper
- 1 tbsp. olive oil

Instructions:

1. Preheat the oven to 350°F. Lightly grease a baking pan.
2. Combine red onion, cauliflower, olive oil, mushroom, apple cider vinegar, lemon juice, salt, and pepper in a bowl. Mix well.
3. Pour the mixture into the greased baking pan.
4. Place inside the oven and bake for 45 minutes. Stir.
5. When vegetables are golden brown and tender, remove from the oven.
6. Garnish with green onions. Serve and enjoy.

Fresh Asparagus Salad

Ingredients:

- 1/3 cup of hazelnuts
- 4 cups arugula
- 1 tsp. ground pepper
- 4 tsp. lemon juice
- 2 tbsp. sea salt
- virgin olive oil
- 2 lbs. asparagus

Instructions:

1. Preheat the oven to 400°F.
2. Place hazelnuts on a baking tray with parchment paper. Place in the oven for 7 minutes.
3. Transfer hazelnuts to a plate. Optionally, to remove the skins, wrap the nuts in a towel and rub them vigorously.
4. Chop hazelnuts coarsely.
5. Remove the hard ends of the asparagus.
6. Place the stalks on the baking sheet you've used for the hazelnuts. Sprinkle 1 tbsp. olive oil and 1/2 tsp. of salt.
7. Bake for 8 minutes.
8. In a mixing bowl, combine pepper, salt, olive oil, and lemon juice. Mix well.

9. Place the arugula in a medium bowl. Drizzle ½ of the dressing over the veggies. Toss until everything is well coated.
10. Place arugula onto a platter.
11. Arrange asparagus on top. Sprinkle peeled hazelnuts on top.

Detox Bowl

Ingredients:

- 1/2 cup onion, diced
- 1-1/2 tbsp. olive oil or coconut oil
- 1 tbsp. ginger, grated
- 1 tsp. whole mustard seeds
- 1 tsp. turmeric
- 1/2 tsp. cumin
- 1/2 tsp. coriander
- 1/2 tsp. curry powder, add more for taste
- 3/4 tsp. kosher salt
- 1/4 lentils, soaked overnight
- 1/2 cup buckwheat, toasted or brown basmati rice, soaked
- 1-1/2 cup water
- 1 cup vegetable broth
- 2 cups vegetables, chopped such as broccoli, carrot, cauliflower, celery, a fennel bulb, and parsnips
- 2 tbsp. cilantro or Italian parsley, chopped
- lemon or lime, squeezed
- 1 tomato, diced

Instructions:

1. Heat up oil on a medium pot over medium-high heat.
2. Saute onion for about 2-3 minutes.

3. Lower heat to medium and add ginger to saute for a few minutes, or until it's fragrant and the color turns golden.
4. Add salt and pepper according to your taste. Stir and leave to toast for a few more minutes.
5. Put lentils and buckwheat or rice, followed by water, broth, and the remaining vegetables. Bring to a boil and cover.
6. Reduce heat to low and leave to simmer for about 20 minutes. Check every now and then for doneness.
7. Leave to cook for 5-10 minutes more if needed.
8. For a porridge-like consistency, pour in more veggie broth.
9. Upon serving, top with tomato and cilantro or parsley. Dash with salt, pepper, and a choice of citrus. Drizzle olive oil if desired.

Conclusion

Herniated discs can be extremely painful and can lead to a variety of other unpleasant symptoms. It is essential to get a diagnosis made as quickly as possible so that treatment may begin. There are several medical therapies, one of which is surgery, that can assist in the alleviation of pain and the improvement of one's quality of life.

Herniated discs can be a painful illness, but there are several things you can do to control your symptoms, including changing your diet and engaging in physical activity, as well as using other natural remedies. The majority of persons who have herniated discs can experience alleviation from their symptoms with the use of appropriate therapy.

If you suspect that you have a herniated disc, you should make an appointment with a medical professional to acquire a correct diagnosis and treatment plan. In addition to seeking medical attention, you could also find relief from your symptoms by using one or more of the natural treatments described up there. The majority of persons who have herniated discs can experience alleviation from their symptoms with the use of appropriate therapy.

References and Helpful Links

Admin. (2014, January 2). Diet for a herniated disc – heal through nutrition. Priority Health. https://www.priorityhealthyorkville.com/diet-for-a-herniated-disc-heal-through-nutrition/.

administrator. (2021, March 30). Foods to improve herniated discs. CORDUS United States. https://cordus.us/foods-to-improve-herniated-discs-2/.

Devil's claw information | mount sinai—New york. (n.d.). Mount Sinai Health System. Retrieved October 16, 2022, from https://www.mountsinai.org/health-library/herb/devils-claw.

Herniated disc – symptoms, causes, prevention and treatments. (n.d.). Retrieved October 16, 2022, from https://www.aans.org/en/Patients/Neurosurgical-Conditions-and-Treatments/Herniated-Disc.

Herniated disk: Causes, symptoms, diagnosis, and treatment. (2022, February 15). https://www.medicalnewstoday.com/articles/191979.

Herniated disk: What it is, diagnosis, treatment & outlook. (n.d.). Cleveland Clinic. Retrieved October 16, 2022, from https://my.clevelandclinic.org/health/diseases/12768-herniated-disk.

Mayo Foundation for Medical Education and Research. (2022, February 8). Herniated disk. Mayo Clinic. Retrieved October 16, 2022, from https://www.mayoclinic.org/diseases-conditions/herniated-disk/diagnosis-treatment/drc-20354101.

MD, R. S. (n.d.). Epidural steroid injection pain relief success rates. Spine-Health. Retrieved October 16, 2022, from https://www.spine-health.com/treatment/injections/epidural-steroid-injection-pain-relief-success-rates.

The most effective methods of treating lumbar disc with nutrition | Dr. Alireza Sheikhi | 2020) . دکتر علیرضا شیخی, October 5). The Most Effective Methods of Treating Lumbar Disc with Nutrition | Dr. Alireza Sheikhi | دکتر علیرضا شیخی. https://www.drsheikhi.com/content/en/520/Treatment-of-lumbar-disc-with-nutrition.

www.ingramcontent.com/pod-product-compliance
Lightning Source LLC
LaVergne TN
LVHW051924060526
838201LV00062B/4672